The Truth About Diabetes!

Coach Isabelle Yang CNC, NEP

Stephanie Baker-Jones IRNPA

1.5 Contact Hours of Continuing Education

CEP #14982

The Truth About Diabetes

Objectives:

- Participants will be able to articulate how the body gains nutrients and the mechanisms to create and store energy.
- Participants will be able to articulate why blood sugar management is important, the behaviors that lead to blood sugar dysfunction, and the negative results of blood sugar mismanagement.
- Participants will be able to articulate consequences surrounding systemic malfunctions related to blood sugar/insulin processes – specifically diabetes Type 2 and Insulin resistance (IR).
- Participants will be able to articulate steps to identify stages of Diabetes.
- Participants will be able to articulate strategies to prevent diabetes T2, and insulin resistance.

The real story about Diabetes

From the time that I was young my "candy & sweets" were restricted by aunts and other relatives with the warning that If I ate too much sugar I would be on the road to "sugar diabetes"! The people believed that if they avoided what they recognized as "sugar" they were doing work to combat or prevent diabetes. If it were that simple, we wouldn't have a national crisis.

The way to combat this epidemic is to break it down, understand it, and tell you how to prevent it if you don't have it, and how to reverse it if you do.

____

____

____

____

____

How do we gain/create energy?

The body uses three main nutrients to function – carbohydrate, protein, and fat. These nutrients are digested into simpler compounds. Carbohydrates are specifically tasked with energy production and are the main nutrient used for energy (glucose) acquisition. Fats are also used for energy after they are broken into fatty acids. The glucose from carbs is converted into the energy your brain and muscles need to function. Fats and protein are also necessary for energy, but they're more of a long-term fuel source, while carbohydrates fulfill the body's most immediate energy needs.

____

____

____

____

____

What are Carbohydrates?

Carbohydrates

Similar to the other macronutrients – Proteins & Fats, Carbohydrates are needed in the body daily. This, based on my previous analogy is a macronutrient that you want to have in your nutrition bank.

Carbohydrates are your body's main source of energy: They help fuel your brain, kidneys, heart muscles, and central nervous system. Our body is efficient in that we can store extra carbohydrates in our muscles and liver for use when we are not getting enough carbohydrates in our diet. Choosing nutrient-dense healthy carbohydrates.

A carbohydrate – deficient diet may cause headaches, fatigue weakness, difficulty concentrating, nausea, constipation, bad breath and vitamin and mineral deficiencies.

____

____

____

____

____

There are three types of carbohydrates (Triplets) and we are going to look at each one.

Sugars – The building block of sugars and starches is the single sugar molecule known as a monosaccharide.

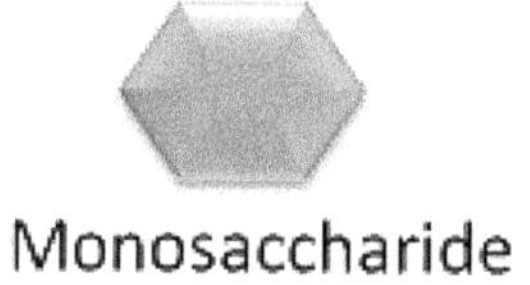

Monosaccharide

Simple=Natural (vegetables, fruits, milk & honey)

One (monosaccharide) sugar molecule - Glucose, galactose, and fructose.

Two (disaccharide) sugar molecules - Lactose, Maltose, and sucrose

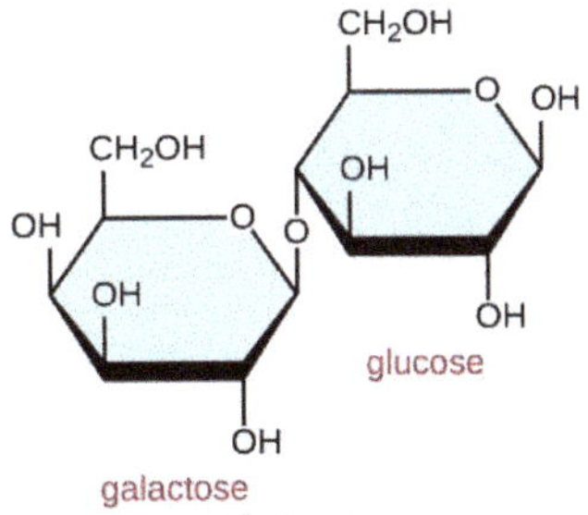

CH_2OH OH OH CH_2OH OH O O OH OH OH glucose OH galactose

lactose

Added (processed foods, syrups, sugary drinks, and candy/sweets. You should avoid added sugar, processed foods, refined grains (like white bread), sodas, other sugary drinks, and sweets as much as possible.

Simple carbs are sugars. While some of these occur naturally in milk, most of the simple carbs in the American diet are added to foods.

Common simple carbs added to foods include:

- raw sugar
- brown sugar
- corn syrup and high fructose corn syrup
- glucose, fructose, and sucrose
- fruit juice concentrate

Starches – Many sugar molecules linked together is a polysaccharide. Glycogen = polysaccharides are the storage forms of glucose in plants and animals.

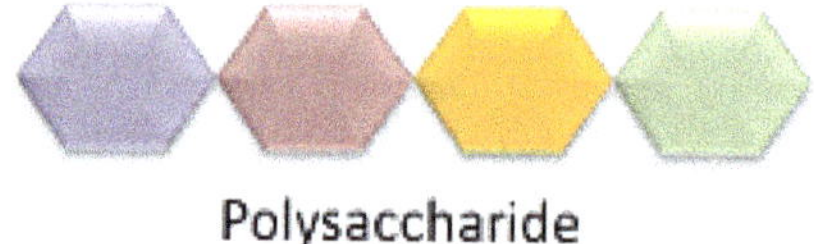

Polysaccharide

Specifically, starch is composed of the sugar **glucose**. Glucose is a sugar molecule made up of carbon ©, hydrogen (H), and oxygen.

Since starch is composed of glucose molecules, the basic formula of starch is very similar to that of glucose. However, in order to link together, glucose molecules have to lose some of their components.

Consider this: If you want to hold hands with someone, you can't be holding anything else. Similarly, the glucose molecule has to empty its hand by letting go of H and O in order to hold hands with another glucose molecule. The H and O are given off as water.

Since starch is made solely of glucose molecules linked together, it is called a **homosaccharide**, a chain of sugars made up of one type of molecule.

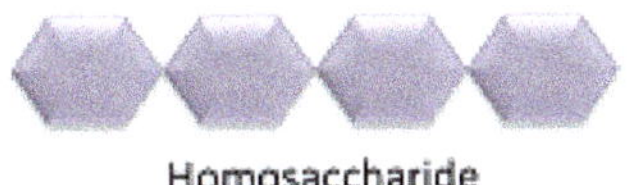
Homosaccharide

Starch is a chain of glucose molecules, but the chain isn't always straight. Sometimes, the sugar molecules branch off from the main chain and form their own, just like a tree has a main trunk and then branches. As such, starch actually has two forms:

one form has no branches – Amylose

while the other form does – Amylopectin

The branchless form is **amylose**.

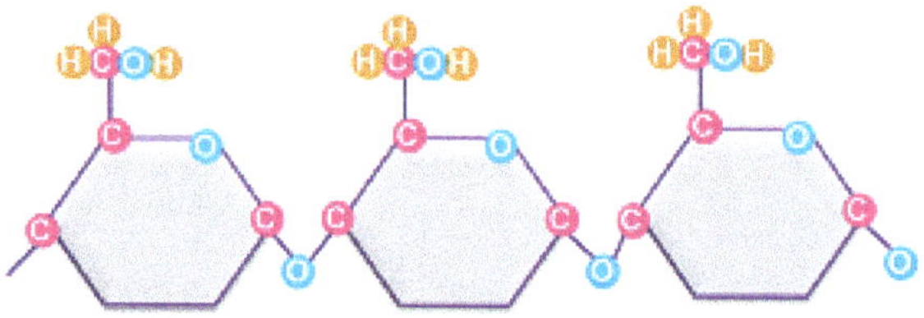

Amylose

Amylose can contain over 250 glucose units per one molecule of amylose.

Amylose can contain over 250 glucoses units per one molecule of amylose. Since it doesn't have branches, amylose can form a 3-D helical structure, much like a slinky. Imagine a completely unwound slinky. It would be awkward to carry around and hard to store. The 'slinky' structure of amylose allows cells to store energy in a compact form, but also makes it easily accessible.

Interestingly, since iodine can insert itself into the helix structure and stains blue, scientists often use iodine to test for the presence of starch.

Amylopectin is the branched form of starch and can contain over 1,000 glucose units. The main chain of hand-holding glucoses is still there, so where does the branching-off glucose attach? It attaches to a different carbon, rather like a third person holding on to your belt while you hold hands with two other people.

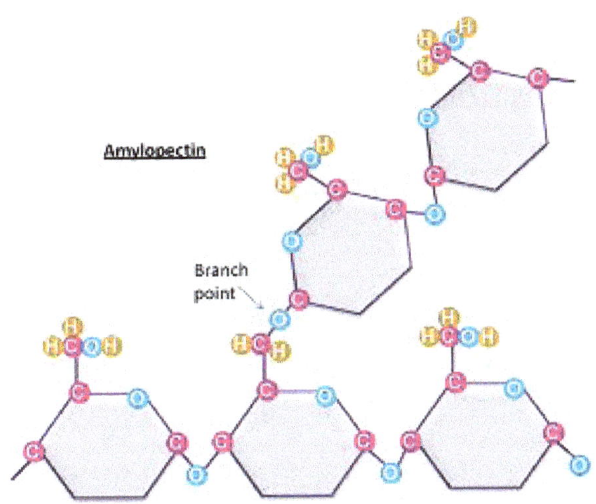

Amylopectin

About every 20 to 25 glucose molecules, a branch point occurs where one molecule of glucose decides to go off in a different direction.

Starch is a chain of glucose molecules, but the chain isn't always straight. Sometimes, the sugar molecules branch off from the main.

Complex - Found in grains, legumes and starchy vegetables such as potatoes and corn.

Starchy foods are an important source of energy. After they are eaten, they are broken down into glucose, which is the body's main fuel, especially for our brain and muscles. Starchy foods provide important nutrients to the diet including B vitamins, iron, calcium and folate.

Fiber – Aids in digestion – helps you feel full and keeps blood cholesterol levels in check.

Dietary fiber is mainly found in fruits, vegetables, whole grains and legumes

Best known for its ability to prevent or relieve constipation the main function is to sweep the colon clean as it exits the body.

My personal favorite reference to fiber- "The broom of the colon!"

Roughage or bulk includes the parts of plant foods your body can't digest or absorb.

Unlike other macronutrients – which your body breaks down and absorbs – fiber isn't digested by our body.

Fiber passes relatively intact through the stomach, small intestine, and colon and out of the body.

Fiber is commonly classified as

Soluble, which dissolves in water.

This type of fiber dissolves in water to form a gel-like material. It can help lower blood cholesterol and glucose levels. Soluble fiber is found in oats, peas, beans, apples, citrus fruits, carrots, barley and psyllium.

Insoluble, which doesn't dissolve in water

This type of fiber promotes the movement of material through your digestive system and increases stool bulk, so it can be of benefit to those who struggle with constipation or irregular stools. Whole-wheat flour, wheat bran, nuts, beans and vegetables, such as cauliflower, green beans and potatoes, are good sources of insoluble fiber.

The amount of soluble and insoluble fiber varies in different plant foods. To receive the greatest health benefit, eat a wide variety of high-fiber foods. Our food is processed in the stomach and broken down into glucose to enter into the blood stream.

____

____

____

____

____

Key Nutrients

1. **Fiber** is found in plant foods that we eat – fruits, grains, legumes and all vegetables. Fiber is essential in slowing down the digestion of carbohydrate, hence, help to release glucose at a

slower and constant rate. The primary functions of fiber is to increase satiety, help to prevent obesity, lower blood glucose levels, normalize bowl movements, lower blood cholesterol levels, decrease risk of cardiovascular disease, and prevent constipation and diverticulosis (Weller, 2007). Recommended intake is between 30 to 50 mg. Transition from low to high fiber diet should be done in increments to avoid gastrointestinal discomfort. Increase fluid intake will help the body to adjust to the increased amount.

2. **Chromium** is a nutrient that is essential for fat and carbohydrate metabolism. It improves glucose tolerance and insulin sensitivity. It's been suggested that a low amount or deficiency of chromium could increase the risk of developing Type II Diabetes (Weller, 2007). A study in 2006 with 1,700 subjects found not only chromium is helpful in supporting healthy blood glucose and insulin levels, but also reduces cholesterol and triglyceride levels (Joval, 2008). Therapeutic dosage of 400 to 800 mcg/day chromium picolinate is recommended to improve glucose tolerance and insulin sensitivity (Bauman, 2012). Best food sources include green peas, green peppers, eggs, beef, onion, and broccoli.

3. **Alpha Lipoic Acid** is an antioxidant that plays a vital role in protecting tissue from oxidative damages causing by high blood sugar level. 20% of diabetes patients develop peripheral neuropathy and 25% develops cardiovascular autonomic neuropathy. Studies have shown that ALA reduces symptoms of diabetic neuropathy and has the ability to increase insulin sensitivity. Recommended dosage is 300 - 600mg/day (Bauman,

2012). Food sources are limited. Very small amount is found in organ meat such as heart, kidney, and liver. Plant sources are from broccoli, spinach, green peas, and tomato.

Additional Nutrient Support

- **L-carnitine** – improves glucose disposal in type 2 diabetic patients
- **L-glutamine** reduces sugar craving, aids in release of insulin
- **Quercetin** – helps protect the membranes of the lens of the eyes from accumulations of polyols
- **Vanadium** – aids insulin's ability to move glucose into the cells; use vanadyl sulfate form
- **Vitamin B complex** – improves metabolism of glucose, energy production, circulation, prevention of atherosclerosis
- **Vitamin C** – Reduces complication arise from oxidative damages

Glucose in the Blood

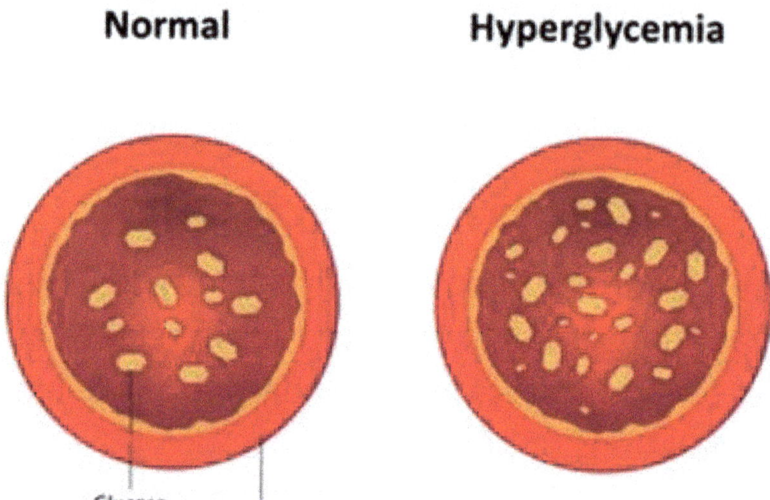

How does the body use glucose?

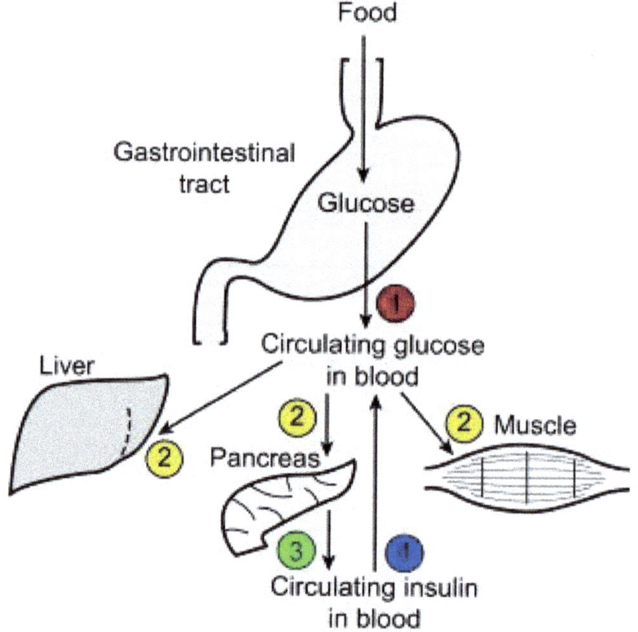

Insulin is the key hormone of carbohydrate metabolism (3). It also influences the metabolism of fats and proteins. It lowers blood glucose by increasing glucose transport in muscle and adipose tissue and stimulates the synthesis of glycogen, fat and protein. Insulin helps glucose enter the body's cells (2) to be used for energy. If all of the glucose is not needed for energy, some of it is stored in fat cells and in the liver as glycogen. As sugar moves from the blood to the cells, the blood glucose level returns to a normal between – meal range (4).

Normal Blood Sugar Cycle

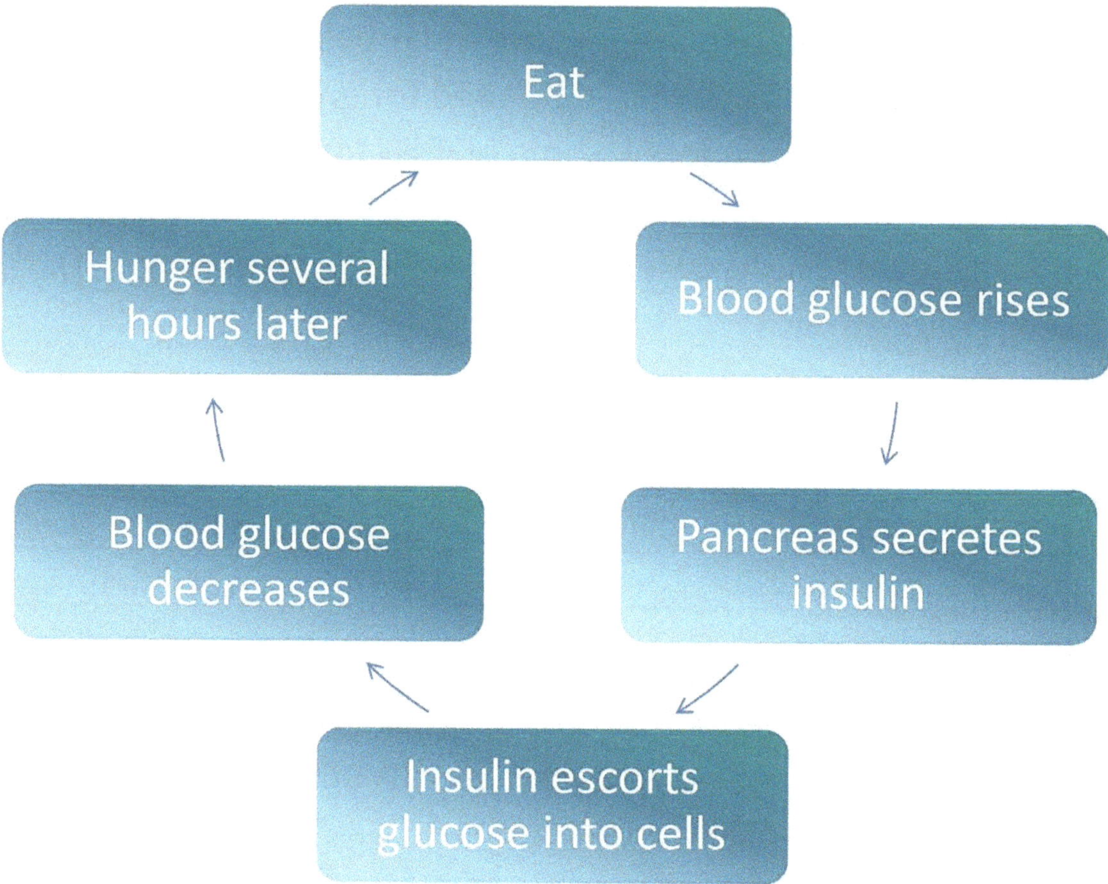

1. Eat
2. Blood glucose rises
3. Pancreas secretes insulin
4. Insulin escorts glucose into cells
5. Blood glucose decreases
6. Hunger several hours later
7. Eat

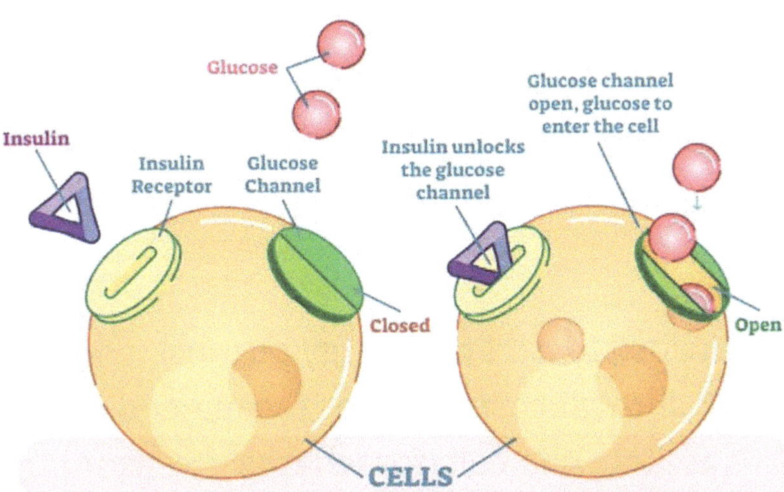

Think of this whole interaction from a social standpoint. Everything breaks down into glucose or fiber. Glucose must get into the cell and the only way to get in is to have an insulin escort. The blood cells work best when the sugar molecules stay within a range. Hemoglobin is the oxygen carrying part of the blood cell and has a life cycle of 3-4 months (100 to 120 days). In the blood stream the glucose molecules attach to the hemoglobin. When systems are working properly the pancreas secretes insulin which meets glucose in the blood stream and the couple enter the cell to be converted to energy.

____

____

____

____

____

What is Diabetes?

Diabetes is much more complicated than avoiding processed sugar. It is about how our bodies process carbohydrates for energy to run all of the bodily processes needed for life.

The cells require glucose (based on energy output), and the food that we eat breaks down into glucose to meet those needs. The excess glucose that can't get into the cell (for whatever reason) begins to cause problems elsewhere.

____

____

____

____

____

Two types of Diabetes

Type 1 – Insulin Dependent Diabetes Mellitis

Sometimes the problems is that there is not enough insulin being made, and in these cases, providing exogenous (outside) insulin is the solution. This describes Type 1 diabetes which is when the body's immune system destroys pancreatic beta cells which are the only cells in the body that make the hormone insulin, which regulates blood glucose. Only about 5% of people with diabetes have this form of the disease. This form is called insulin dependent diabetes mellitis and to survive this lack of insulin production they must have insulin delivered by injection or a pump.

Type 2 – Non-Insulin Dependent Diabetes Mellitis

The pathogenesis (disease beginning) of Type 2 diabetes ordinarily involves the development of insulin resistance associated with compensatory hyperinsulinemia, followed by progressive beta cell impairment that results in decreasing insulin secretion and hyperglycemia.

Type II Diabetes Risk Factors

- **Being overweight** - fatty tissue are resistant to insulin
- **Fat distribution** – fat stored primarily in the abdomen
- **Lack of physical activity** – being active help with weight and usage of glucose as energy and makes your cells more sensitive to insulin
- **Family history** –increase risk if parents or sibling has type 2 diabetes
- **Race** – blacks, Hispanics, American Indians and Asian-Americans
- **Age** over 45
- **Prediabetes** – blood sugar higher than normal, but not enough to be classified as diabetes.
- **Gestation diabetes** – pregnancy induced diabetes and/or giving birth to a baby weighting more than 9 pounds

Nutritional Causes of Diabetes

- Omega-3 fat DHA deficiency
- Elevated omega-6 – omega-3 fat
- Trans fats
- Deficiencies of chromium, magnesium, zinc, B vitamins, boron, and lithium
- Eating high-glycemic meals, snacks, and sweet drinks
- Insufficient protein

Lab Marker Patterns

	Normal	Insulin Resistance	Metabolic Syndrome	Diabetes
Fasting Glucose	75-89	90-119	>=100	>=120
Triglycerides	>65	>90	>110	>110
HDL	50-90	<65	<55	<55
Fasting Insulin	2-5	Normal or >5 – varies on stage	>5	>5
Hemoglobin A1C	4.5 – 5%	5.3-6.5%	>5.7%	>5.7%

A normal A1C level is below 5.7%, a level of 5.7 % - 6.4% indicates prediabetes, and a level of 6.5% or more indicates diabetes. Within the 5.7 % to 6.4% prediabetes range, the higher you're a1C, the greater your risk is for developing type 2 diabetes.

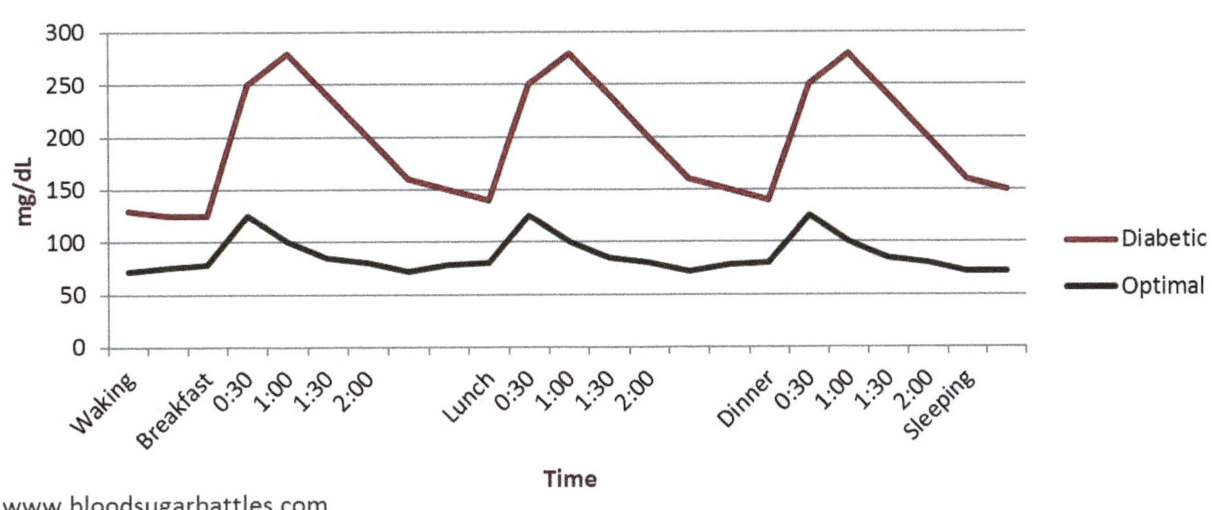

Diabetes is on the rise: 422 million adults have diabetes. 3.7 million deaths are due to diabetes and high blood glucose. 1.5 million deaths are caused by diabetes. That works out to be: one (1) person in 11.

____

____

____

____

____

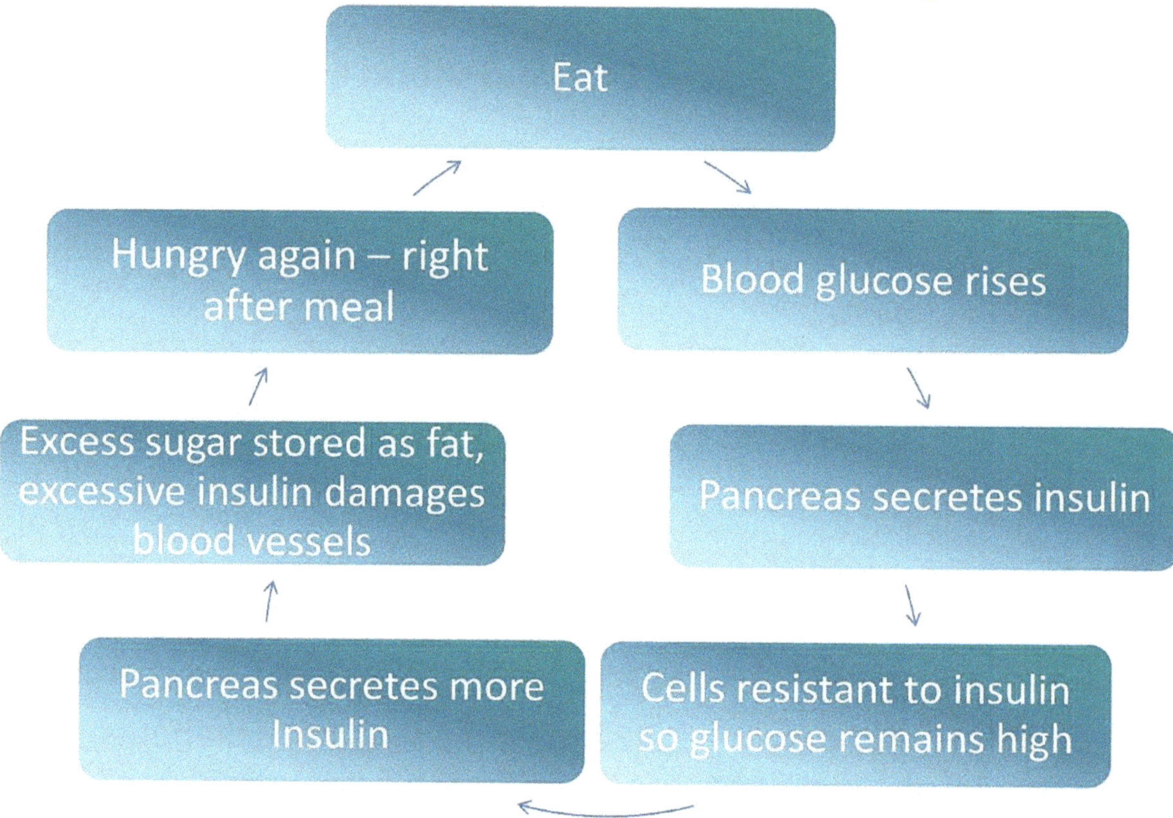

1. Eat
2. Blood glucose rises
3. Pancreas secretes insulin
4. Cells resistant to insulin so glucose remains high
5. Pancreas secretes more insulin
6. Excess sugar stored as fat, excessive insulin damages blood vessels
7. Hungry again – right after meal
8. Eat

Stressors that Trigger Blood Sugar Response

- Mental and emotional stress
- Digestive imbalance: leaky gut, candida, parasites
- Inflammation
- Food stress: nutrient depleted foods high in toxic, high-glycemic foods
- Obesity
- Immune system imbalance
- Injuries
- Toxic exposure
- Sleep quality and quantity
- Eating too close to bedtime

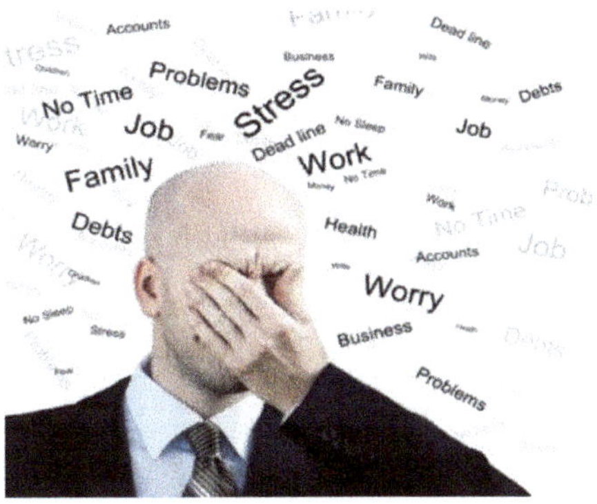

Leading complications of Diabetes

- Heart disease/Hypertension – 68%
- Nervous system disease/Amputations – 60%
- Eye problems leading to blindness – 28%
- Complications of Pregnancy – 20%
- Dental Disease – 9%

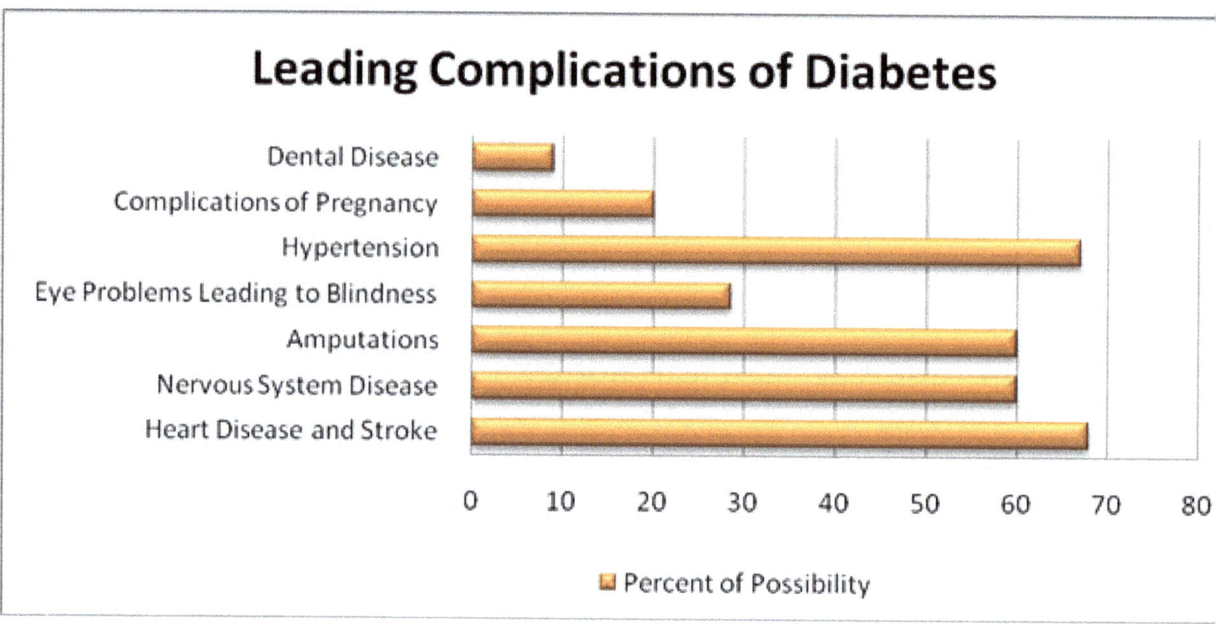

Causes of Insulin Resistance

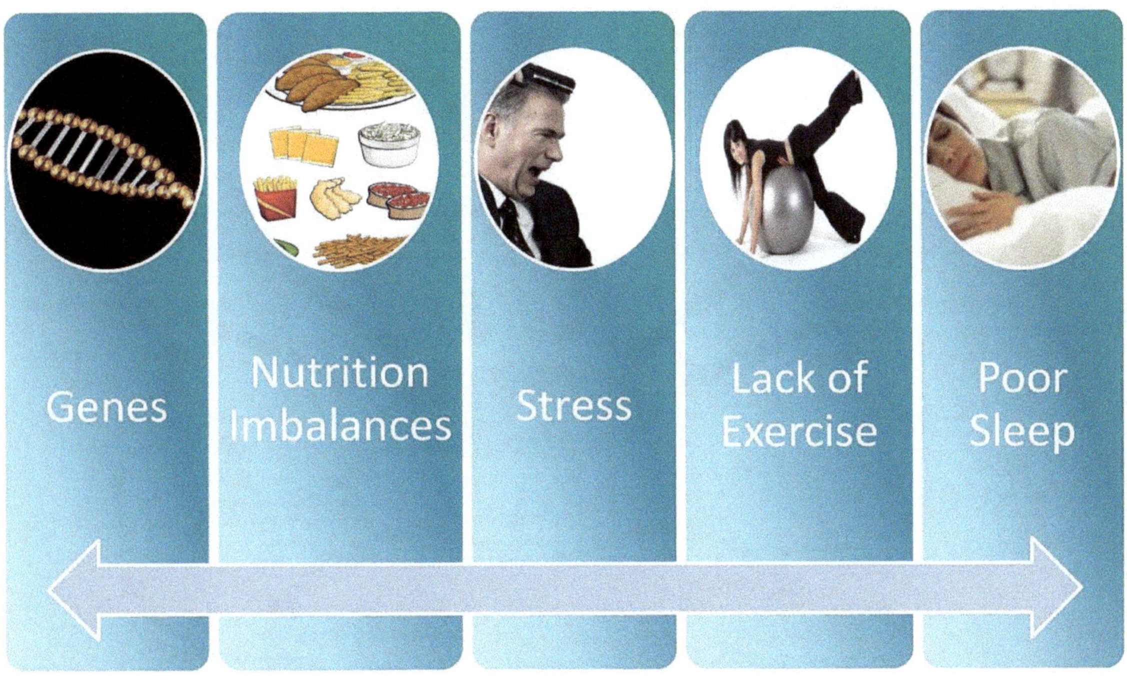

- Belly fat
- Low energy especially after meals
- Hungry even after a full meal
- Mid-afternoon energy slump
- Difficulty focusing
- Cranky and irritable if meal missed

____

____

____

____

____

Symptoms of Insulin Resistance

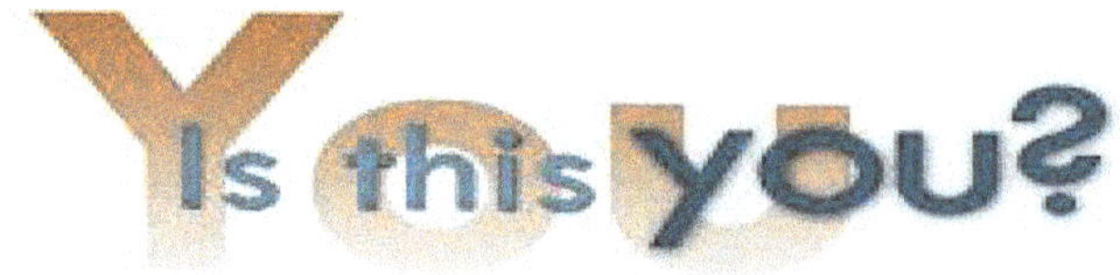

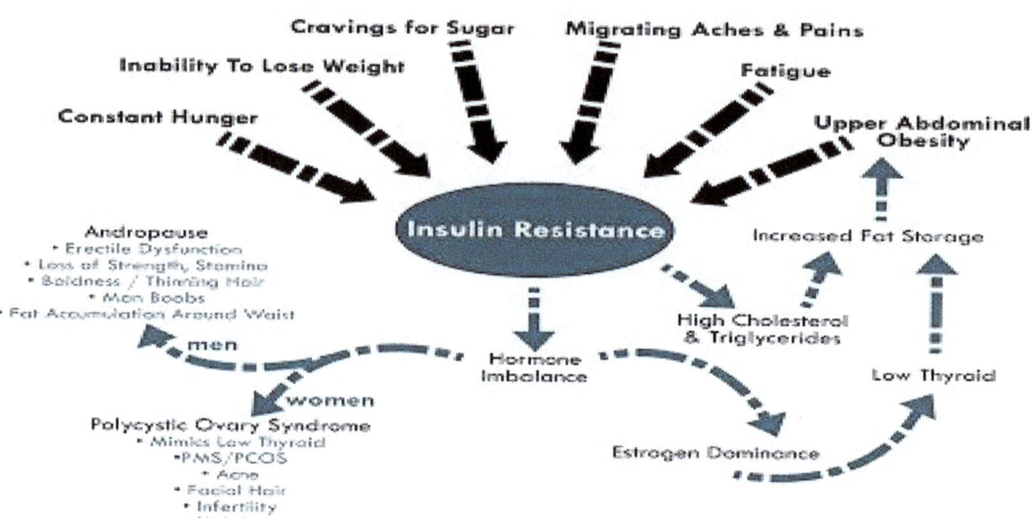

- Constant hunger
- Inability to lose weight
- Cravings for Sugar
- Migrating Aches & Pains
- Fatigue
- Upper Abdominal Obesity

____

____

____

____

____

The Serious Consequences of Insulin Resistance

- Thyroid and growth hormone deficiency
- Increased cancer risk
- High blood pressure
- Injury to blood vessel linings
- Systemic inflammation
- Risk of Alzheimer's
- Low energy in all organs and glands
- Diabetes

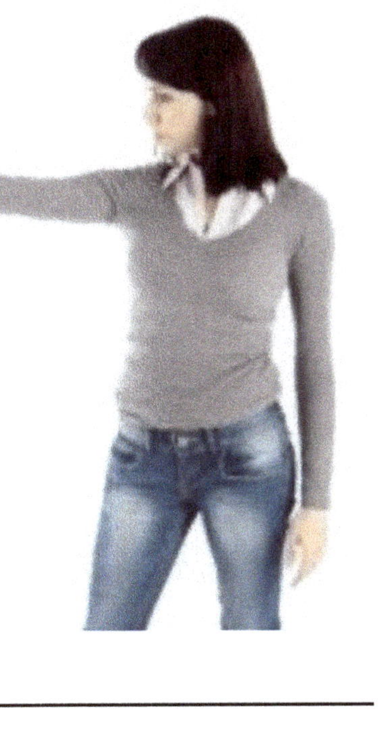

6 Steps to Reverse Insulin Resistance

1. Movement – strength training and high intensity burst exercises are most efficient in reversing insulin resistance.
2. Eat Right: Green and Sea vegetables, Avocado, Chia seeds, Cinnamon, Ginger. Reduce high carbohydrate foods including whole grains and fruits high in glycemic index.
3. Relax – Constant high stress situation or mindset causes the body to produce cortisol which signals the body to raise and keep glucose level high.
4. Sleep More and Early – Many hormones are produced while we sleep for example DHEA. DHEA helps to regulate blood sugar and increase our body's insulin sensitivity.
5. Stop Snacking – frequent snacking means your pancreas is constantly required to produce insulin to move glucose into the bloodstream. This increases the likelihood of your cells becoming resistant to insulin and high glucose in the bloodstream which may damage the epithelial lining of your arteries.
6. Banish Toxins – toxins disruptions cellular function and There Is no Organ System in our bodies that is immune to the effects of toxicity in the environment

____

____

____

____

____

Blood sugar dysregulation is the culprit to chronic illnesses

Here are: The 7 leading causes of death in the U.S.

- Heart disease
- Cancer
- Chronic lower respiratory disease
- Stroke
- Accidents
- Alzheimer's disease
- Diabetes

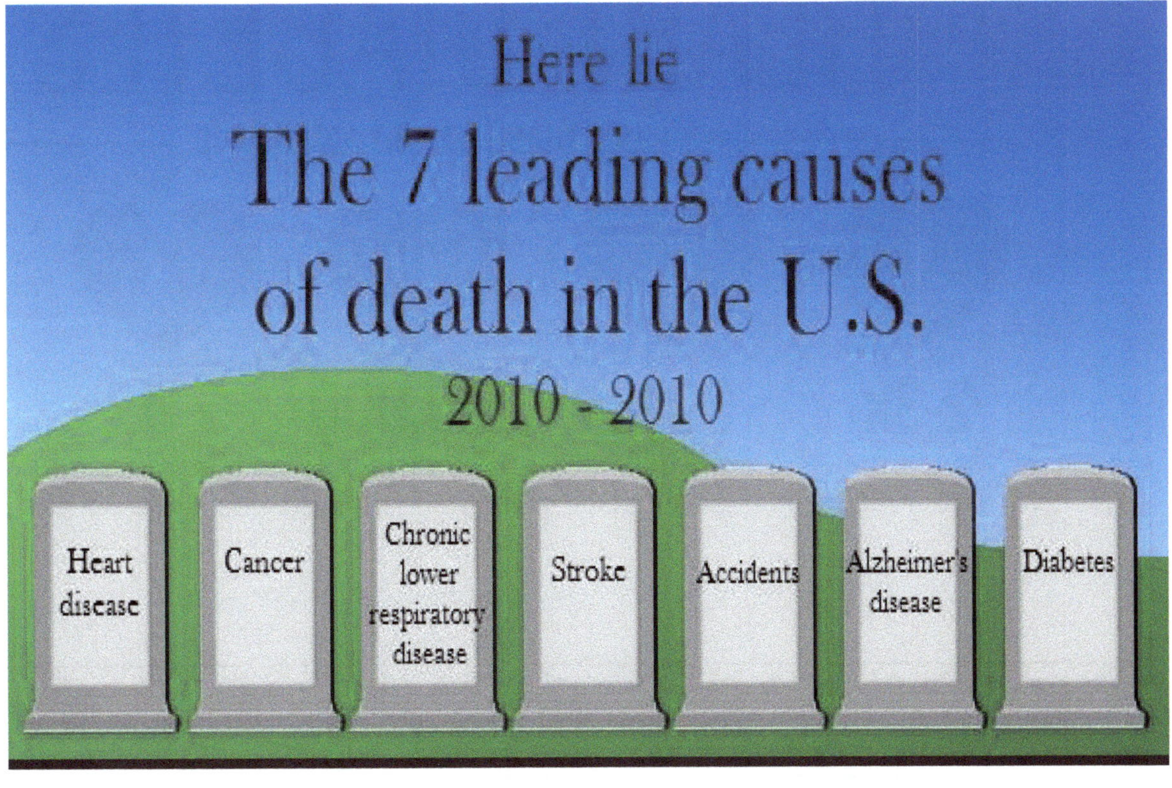

____

____

____

____

____

Diabetes and Heart Disease

U.S. Diabetes patients

- 2-3 times the increased risk for heart disease
- 30% more coronary (heart) stents implanted in 2011
- 280,000 heart attacks annually
- 2 – 4 times higher heart disease morbidity and mortality rates
- 60% chance of dying from heart disease.

AT THE HEART OF DIABETES

Diabetes & Heart Disease By The #s

U.S. DIABETES PATIENTS HAVE:

2-3x increased risk for heart disease

30% of coronary stents implanted in 2011

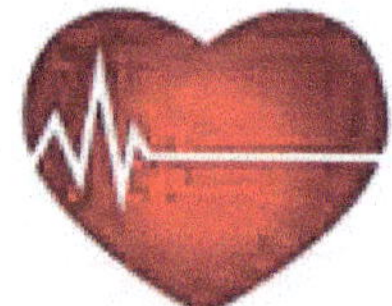

280,000 heart attacks annually

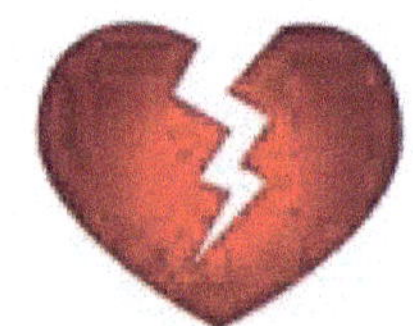

2-4x higher heart disease morbidity and mortality rates

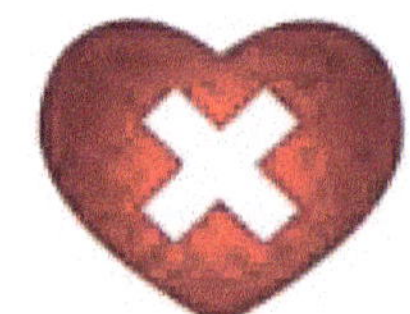

60% chance of dying from heart disease

Post-Test/Assessment

1. How does the body gain nutrients?

____
____
____
____
____

2. How does the body create energy?

____
____
____
____
____

3. How does the body store energy?

____
____
____
____
____

4. Why is blood sugar management important?

____
____
____
____
____

5. What behaviors lead to blood sugar dysfunction?

____
____
____
____
____

6. What are the results of blood sugar mismanagement?

____
____
____
____
____

7. What are the consequences of Type 2 diabetes?

____
____
____
____
____

8. What are the consequences of insulin resistance?

____
____
____
____
____

9. What are the stages of diabetes?

____
____
____
____
____

10. What are the strategies to prevent diabetes Type 2?

____
____
____
____
____

11. What are the strategies to prevent insulin resistance?

____
____
____
____
____

12. Can you reverse diabetes? (circle one)

YES NO

13. Why or why not?

____
____
____

14. What strategies would you implement?

The Truth About Diabetes

Evaluation (1.5 Contact Hours (CH) will be awarded)

Name of Participant________________________________ Title________________

License/Certification #________________________________ Exp. Date___________

Date Completed: ____________________________

For the following questions answer: 1)-No agreement, 2)-Some agreement, 3)-Moderate agreement, 4)-High agreement, 5)-Not Applicable

The objectives and content of the program were relevant to my needs as a healthcare provider.

1 2 3 4 5

The presenters were knowledgeable and well prepared.

1 2 3 4 5

The presentation was clear and logical.

1 2 3 4 5

I will be able to apply the knowledge or skills gained in my healthcare practice.

1 2 3 4 5

The format was conducive to the education process.

1 2 3 4 5

How will you implement this content to empower the clients that you encounter in your healthcare practice?

____

____

____

____

____

I would recommend this program to colleagues. (circle one)

Yes No

____

____

____

____

____

Comments/Suggestions:

____

____

____

____

____

This evaluation and post-test will be retained with the CE provider along with a copy of the certificate issued.

Healthcare Professionals only!

To submit: email post-test and evaluation: C4lCEP@gmail.com

Subject: Diabetes CE

LE-AL Productions R.E.A.L. Knowledge CEP#14982/Healthy Gut Vibrant Life

Submit 30.00 (US) payment to: Paypal.me/sbaker396

CE certificate for 1.5 CH will be emailed back to you

Please write legibly and complete all forms

Post-test will be corrected and returned.

Thank you for your patronage!

Get your certificate of completion – No continuing education contact hours

COMPLIMENTARY!

Non-Healthcare Professionals!

To submit: email post-test and evaluation: C4lCEP@gmail.com

Subject: Diabetes Class

LE-AL Productions R.E.A.L. Knowledge/Healthy Gut Vibrant Life

Completion certificate will be emailed back to you

Please write legibly and complete all forms (N/A for licensure# /expiration date

Post-test will be corrected and returned

Thank you for your patronage!

REFERENCES

Bauman, E, 2011. NC206.03 Lecture – Diabetes: Type I & II. Retrieved from Bauman College: http://dashboard.baumancollege.org/pluginfile.php/3610/mod_resource/content/5/TN_Materials/206/Lecture/unzip206.03/player.html

Bauman, E. Friedlander, J. (2011). Therapeutic Nutrition. Penngrove, CA:Bauman College

Packer, L., & Colman, C. (1999). The *antioxidant miracle.* New York, NY: John Wiley & Sons, Inc.

Joval, S.Joval, S. (with Mitchell, D.). (2008). *What Your Doctor May Not Tell You About Diabetes: An Innovative Program to Prevent, Treat, and Beat This Controllable Disease*. New York, New York:Grand Central Publishing

Weller P. (2007). *The Power of Nutrient Dense Food*. California:Deerpath Publishing Company

www.ingramcontent.com/pod-product-compliance
Ingram Content Group UK Ltd.
Pitfield, Milton Keynes, MK11 3LW, UK
UKHW050148280726
14058UKWH00007B/889